INSIGHT ON PANCREATIC CANCER:

Causes, Symptoms, Effects, And Treatment.

By

PRISCILLA HUNT

Table of content

INTRODUCTION:

A kind of cancer called pancreatic   cancer

develops in the pancreas, an organ beneath the stomach. It happens when pancreatic cells start to multiply uncontrolled and form a tumor. Since pancreatic cancer is frequently discovered in an advanced stage, effective treatment is challenging. Abdominal pain, jaundice (skin and eye yellowing), weight loss, and digestive issues are typical symptoms. Depending on the stage and severity of the cancer, treatment options may include surgery, chemotherapy, radiation therapy, or a combination of these.

Although there is a relatively low survival rate for this dangerous and sometimes aggressive cancer, early detection, and immediate medical care can improve prognosis.

Chapter 1

What is pancreatic cancer?

The pancreas is an organ in your abdomen that is located behind the bottom portion of your stomach. Pancreatic cancer starts in the tissues of the pancreas. Your pancreas generates hormones that help you control your blood sugar as well as enzymes that help with digestion.

The pancreas can develop both malignant and noncancerous tumors, among other growths. Pancreatic ductal adenocarcinoma, the most prevalent form of pancreatic cancer, develops in the cells that line the ducts that remove digestive enzymes from the pancreas.

Rarely is pancreatic cancer found in its earliest stages, when it is most treatable. This is due to the fact that symptoms frequently don't appear until the disease has spread to other organs.

Options for treating pancreatic cancer are

determined

Depending on how far advanced the illness is, many treatments are available for pancreatic cancer. Surgery, chemotherapy, radiation therapy, or a combination of these are all possible options.

Your pancreas measures around 6 inches (15 cm) in length and resembles a pear that has been turned on its side. To assist your body in metabolizing the sugar in the meals you eat, it releases (secretes) hormones like insulin.

Additionally, it creates digestive fluids to aid in food digestion and nutritional absorption.

Genesis of pancreatic cancer

When cells in your pancreas experience DNA changes (mutations), pancreatic cancer results. The instructions that inform a cell what to do are encoded in its DNA. The cells are instructed by these mutations to grow uncontrollably and to live on after normal cells expire. These accumulating cells have the potential to create a tumor.

Pancreatic cancer cells can spread to surrounding organs and blood vessels, as well as distant sections of the body, if left untreated.

The majority of pancreatic cancers arise in the cells that border the pancreatic ducts. This is known as pancreatic adenocarcinoma or pancreatic exocrine cancer. Cancer can arise in the pancreas' hormone-producing cells or neuroendocrine cells less commonly. These cancers are known as pancreatic neuroendocrine tumors, islet cell tumors, or pancreatic endocrine tumors.

Chapter 2: Pancreatic Cancer Causes

Pancreatic Cancer is caused by changes in your DNA. These can be passed on from your parents or developed over time. Changes that occur over time may occur as a result of being exposed to something toxic. They can also occur at random.

The specific causes of pancreatic cancer remain unknown. About 10% of pancreatic cancers are inherited.

Other risk factors that enhance your chances of developing

pancreatic cancer include:

1. Smoking
2. Diabetes Pancreatitis
3. Chronic inflammation of the pancreas
4. Pancreatic cancer in the family
5. Obesity

6. Older age, as the majority of patients are diagnosed after the age of 65.

The combination of smoking, long-term diabetes, and a poor diet raises the risk of pancreatic cancer above and beyond the risk of any of these factors alone.

Also,

- Red meat may raise the risk of pancreatic cancer.
- Processed meat eating may raise the risk of pancreatic cancer.
- Consumption of saturated fatty acid-containing foods may

raise the risk of pancreatic cancer.

- Alcohol intake may raise the risk of pancreatic cancer.

- Consumption of fructose-containing foods and beverages may raise the risk of pancreatic cancer.

Chapter 3: Effects of Pancreatic Cancer

As pancreatic cancer spreads, it may result in difficulties like:

- **Loss of weight**.
People with pancreatic cancer may lose weight for a variety of reasons. As the body's energy is used up by the malignancy, weight loss may occur. It could be challenging to eat due to nausea and vomiting

brought on by cancer therapies or a tumor pressing against your stomach. Or perhaps your pancreas isn't producing enough digestive fluids, which prevents your body from properly absorbing nutrients from food.

- **Jaundice**:

Jaundice can be brought on by pancreatic cancer that restricts the liver's bile duct. Yellow skin and eyes, dark urine, and light-colored feces are symptoms. To keep the bile duct open, your doctor may advise implanting a plastic or metal tube (stent). This is accomplished through a technique known as endoscopic retrograde cholangiopancreatog raphy. During ERCP, an endoscope is inserted into the top portion of your small intestine after being inserted down your throat, and through your stomach. A tiny hollow tube (catheter) is then inserted through the endoscope into the pancreatic and bile ducts to inject a dye.

Finally, pictures of the ducts are taken.

- **Pain**: Your abdomen's nerves may become compressed when a tumor grows, resulting in potentially life-threatening agony. Painkillers may make you feel more at ease. Radiation and chemotherapy treatments may be able to reduce discomfort and inhibit the growth of the tumor.

In severe cases, your doctor may advise a surgery called a celiac plexus block, which involves injecting alcohol into the nerves that regulate your abdominal pain. This technique prevents your brain from receiving pain signals from your nerves.

•**Intestine blockage**: The movement of digested food from your stomach into your intestines can be obstructed by pancreatic cancer that invades or presses on the duodenum, the first segment of the small intestine.

Your physician might advise having a tube (stent) put inside your small intestine to keep it open. In certain cases, surgery to insert a temporary feeding tube or join your stomach to a lower area in your intestines that isn't obstructed by cancer may be beneficial.

Chapter 4: Types of Pancreatic cancer

There are various cancer kinds in each group, and their symptoms and prognosis can vary.

1. Exocrine pancreatic cancer, which includes adenocarcinoma

2. neuroendocrine pancreatic cancer

are the two main subtypes of pancreatic cancer.

Pancreatic Cancer: Exocrine (Nonendocrine)

Exocrine cells, which make up the exocrine gland and ducts of the pancreas, are the source of exocrine pancreatic cancer. In the duodenum, the exocrine gland secretes enzymes that aid in the breakdown of carbs, lipids, proteins, and acids.

More than 95% of all pancreatic cancers are different kinds of exocrine pancreatic cancer. These are a few of them:

- **Adenocarcinoma**

Adenocarcinoma, also known as ductal carcinoma, is the most prevalent form of pancreatic cancer, making up more than 90% of all diagnoses. This cancer develops in the pancreatic duct lining.

The cells that produce pancreatic enzymes may also grow into adenocarcinomas.

Acinar cell carcinoma, which makes up about 1% to 2% of exocrine malignancies, when that happens.

Adenocarcinoma symptoms, such as nausea, weight loss, and stomach pain, are similar to those of acinar cell carcinoma. Jaundice is less typical, though. Some people may experience skin rashes and joint pain as a result of an increase in enzymes.

- **Cancer of the Squamous Cells**: This exceedingly rare pancreatic nonendocrine cancer consists entirely of squamous cells, which are not commonly found in the pancreas. It develops in the pancreatic ducts. The roots of this disease are not entirely understood because there are not enough reported cases of it. The majority of cases are first detected after metastasis, according to studies, giving it an extremely poor prognosis.

• **Acromegalic Carcinoma**

One percent to four percent of exocrine pancreatic cancers are this uncommon form of the disease. Adenosquamous carcinoma is a more aggressive tumor with a worse prognosis than adenocarcinoma. These tumors have traits common to squamous cell carcinoma and ductal adenocarcinoma.

- **Colloid Cancer:** Colloid carcinomas, another uncommon form, make up 1% to

3% of exocrine pancreatic malignancies. These tumors typically arise from an intraductal papillary mucinous neoplasm (IPMN), a specific kind of benign cyst. The pancreatic colloid tumor is less likely to spread and is simpler to treat than other pancreatic tumors because it is made up of malignant cells that float on a gelatinous material called mucin. Additionally, the prognosis is significantly better.

PANCREATIC NEUROENDOC RINE CANCER

Cells in the pancreatic endocrine gland, which secretes the chemicals insulin and glucagon into the bloodstream to regulate blood sugar, give rise to pancreatic neuroendocrine tumors. Neuroendocrine malignancies, also known as endocrine or islet cell tumors, are uncommon, accounting for fewer than 5% of all cancers.

The rare forms of cancer called pancreatic neuroendocrine tumors begin as cell proliferation in the pancreas. Behind the stomach, the pancreas is a long, flat gland. It produces hormones and enzymes that aid in food digestion.

The pancreatic hormone-producing cells are the origin of

pancreatic neuroendocrine tumors. Islet cells are the name for these cells. Islet cell carcinoma is another name for pancreatic neuroendocrine tumors.

Hormone production continues in some pancreatic neuroendocrine tumor cells. The term "functional tumors" refers to these. Functional tumors overproduce the particular hormone. The tumor types insulinoma, gastrinoma, and glucagonoma are examples of functional tumors.

The majority of pancreatic neuroendocrine tumors do not overproduce hormones. Nonfunctional tumors are those that don't create additional hormones.

Symptoms

Sometimes pancreatic neuroendocrine tumors go unnoticed. Symptoms when this occurs can include:

- Heartburn.
- Weakness
- Fatigue.
- Muscle pain.
- Indigestion.
- Diarrhea.

- Loss of weight.
- A skin rash.

- Constipation.
- Back or abdominal pain.
- The whites of the eyes and skin become yellow.
- Dizziness.
- Hazy vision.
- Headaches.

- More hunger and thirst.

Causes

When pancreatic cells experience DNA alterations, pancreatic neuroendocrine tumors result. The instructions that inform a cell what to do are stored in its DNA. The adjustments, which scientists refer to as mutations, instruct the cells to divide quickly. When healthy cells would naturally expire as a part of their life cycle, the alterations allowed the cells to live on. Numerous additional cells are produced as a result. The cells may gather into a mass known as a tumor.

Cells can sometimes separate and travel to other organs, such as the liver. Metastatic cancer occurs when cancer spreads.

The DNA alterations in pancreatic neuroendocrine tumors occur in hormone-producing cells called islet cells. It is unknown what causes the alterations that lead to cancer.

Chapter Five: Treatment for pancreatic cancer

Pancreatic cancer treatment may involve

1. Surgery
2. Chemotherapy
3. Radiation therapy,

4. Vaccination,

5. Pain management

6. Immunotherapy

7. Dietary changes.

About 20% of people with pancreatic cancer have access to **surgery**, which has the potential to be a successful treatment. When surgery is not an option, stereotactic body radiation therapy may be used to treat early-stage pancreatic cancer. If the cancer is localized within the pancreas and has not metastasized (spread) to blood vessels, lymph nodes, or other organs, surgery can be done as a potentially curative therapy. Only around 20% of pancreatic cancer patients, according to the American Society of Clinical Oncology, are candidates for this procedure.

Most pancreatic cancer patients already have metastatic disease at the time of diagnosis. The surgical excision of their primary tumor would not be beneficial for these people. Surgery can, however, be performed to treat symptoms or avoid complications in metastatic cancer patients.

The sort of procedure used to remove

pancreatic cancer depends on the stage and location of the tumor for surgical candidates.

A PATIENT WITH PANCREATIC CANCER CAN HAVE DIFFERENT TYPES OF SURGERY.

Pancreatic Surgery With Little To No Incision

Depending on where the tumor is located, minimally invasive or laparoscopic surgical methods may occasionally be used in pancreatic surgery. Small abdominal incisions are used during laparoscopic surgeries to insert telescope-guided devices.

In traditional procedures, the abdomen must be opened larger and with a longer incision. Surgeons are typically able to minimize the patient's risk of infection and blood loss during laparoscopic procedures. If you are a candidate for a minimally invasive procedure, your surgical oncologist can assist in making that determination.

Transverse Pancreatectomy: A

distal pancreatectomy involves the removal of the pancreas body and tail while keeping the organ's head intact. The spleen is typically also removed.

A Complete Pancreatectomy

This method is done when cancers spread throughout the pancreas and is the least frequent type of pancreatic cancer surgery. The complete pancreas, spleen, gallbladder, common bile duct, as well as a piece of the small intestine and stomach, are all removed during a total pancreatectomy.

After the procedure, the majority of patients will stay in the hospital for one to two weeks. Patients who have had their complete pancreas removed are no longer able to produce either the digestive enzymes or the insulin needed to regulate blood glucose (sugar) levels. Patients are consequently required to take additional enzymes and insulin for the remainder of their lives after surgery.

Surgical Margin:

During surgery, the surgical margins are the edges or borders of the pancreatic cancer tissue that is removed. To ensure that each patient's tumor margins surrounding the surgical excision are assessed during surgery, surgeons and pathologists collaborate.

The pathologist can direct the surgical team toward any lingering cancer cells in the tumor's borderline regions as they are being examined under a microscope in real-time, signaling that more tissue may need to be removed. Some malignant cells cannot always be eradicated.

If a pathologist refers to a margin as "negative" or "clean," it signifies that they did not discover any cancer cells there. If the margin is characterized as positive or involved, it may not have completely eradicated the malignancy.

Surgical Hospice

Surgery may be used to treat or prevent issues like a clogged bile duct or intestine in cases of more advanced malignancy. The goal of palliative surgery is not to treat the condition.

CONCLUSION;

A new vaccination intended to eliminate pancreatic cancer cells is being evaluated in clinical trials. To help maximize comfort and sustain quality of life, a variety of efficient pain management approaches, including pharmaceutical and complementary methods, are available.